Healing The Body & Mind Using Ancestral Knowledge

The Knowledge & Wisdom Of Traditional Healers

Written & Compiled By
Rev. Dr. Geraldine L. Carter

"The natural healing force within each of us is the greatest force in getting well."

-Hippocrates

any usage or abuse of any policies, processes, or directions contained within is the solitary and utter responsibility of the recipient reader. Under no circumstances will any legal responsibility or blame be held against the publisher for any reparation, damages, or monetary loss due to the information herein, either directly or indirectly.

Respective authors own all copyrights not held by the publisher.

The information herein is offered for informational purposes solely, and is universal as so. The presentation of the information is without contract or any type of guarantee assurance.

The trademarks that are used are without any consent, and the publication of the trademark is without permission or backing by the trademark owner. All trademarks and brands within this book are for clarifying purposes only and are then owned by the owners themselves, not affiliated with this document.

Table Of Contents

Introduction

This book is written for those who are interested in the remedies that I found in Belize Central while working on the book Belizean Botanicals and in St. Vincent while working on a book of remedies called Ancestral Healing Remedies.

As a Boonville/Bunceton Missouri girl, I had the opportunity to grow up living in and among healers. But later in my adult life I traveled to Central and South America into the Country of Belize and St. Vincent in the West Indies.

There I lived and studied with Black Carib and Garifuna healers. Many of the remedies I learned that you will read about come from farmers, producers, collectors, herbalists, healers and village women who all have some ideas about plants and foods that can be used as medicine.

It is important for you to know about and use the remedies if you desire, but please do not allow them to serve as a replacement for professional medical care. Listen to your body and pay close attention to how your body reacts to herbs; and adjust your use of them accordingly.

Always use discretion and be aware that the application of home remedies in this book is **AT YOUR OWN RISK**. Not everything will work the same for everyone. The book will be a wonderful reference and resource for those interested in natural healing techniques.

Genesis 1:29-30 states:

And God said "Behold, I have given you every herb bearing seed, which is upon the face of all the earth, and every tree, in which is the fruit of a tree yielding seed; to you, it shall be for meat and to everything wherein there is life, I have given every green herb for meat, and it was so."

Psalms 104:14, which states:

"God caused the grass to grow for the cattle; and herbs, for the service of man."

Revelation 122:2, which states:

"In the midst of the street of it; and on either side of the river, was there the tree of life, which bears twelve manners of fruits, and yielded her fruit every month; and the leaves of the tree were for the healing of nations."

By using the herbs, provided by God for our benefit, we are cooperating with God. In addition to her spiritual practices that were specifically related to God and the Bible, there were also other spiritual practices that related to her success with herbs and healing.

RAINFOREST REMEDIES

Learning From The Rainforest Healers

When I first went to Belize, I fell in love with the country and with the people. I know that my experiences there have greatly enriched my life. It has been my good fortune to be able to spend time with and learn from several folk healers.

These healers greatly expanded my knowledge, acceptance and understanding of ancient spiritual healing. I will go back again not only for the much needed renewal of body and spirit but also to further my studies and to spend more time with folk healers.

My Belizean experiences included encounters with Miss Atillo, Janice Bain and Dr. Macayco. Even though I was aware that there were healers that made use of plants to heal, my great grandmother in Missouri was a practitioner of this art.

I had no real knowledge or exposure to this practice and while I didn't disbelieve I wasn't fully ready to accept it. Miss Atillo opened the door and I began to learn the gentleness and power of healing the old way. Sometime later I encountered Janice Bain.

Her shop and practice Agapi is in Belize City. However, she travels to the country to find her herbs and learns from elder healers. My time with Dr. Macayco in Hopkins Village further opened my mind to the wonders of ancient spiritual healing.

Dr. Macayco was a bit of a character, but then he had every right to be eccentric. It took some time before he would even consider talking with me about herbs and his healing practices and it also took a bottle of rum, but it was worth the wait.

I learned a lot about plants and its uses. With the help of a local teacher and village elders we were able to put a book together of ancient remedies. Most recently I had the opportunity to benefit from the healing of Francisca Ortega.

She is a traditional Kekchi Mayan folk healer in Punta Gorda. On a recent visit to Belize while in the airport shop I found the book, Rainforest Home Remedies, by Rosita Arvigo & Nadine Epstein.

It was the shops last copy of the book and I bought it with my last few Belizean dollars. I was somewhat familiar with the works of Rosita Arvigo but had not had the opportunity to study them in great depth. I spent the plane ride back reading her amazing book.

Rosita Arvigo is a traditional healer, teacher, ethno botanist and doctor of Naprapathy. She is the director of Ix Chel Tropical Research Foundation and founder and co director of Terra Nova, the world's first and only biomedical rainforest reserve.

I'd like to share with you excerpts from Dr. Arvigo's Rainforest Home Remedies, ©Copyright 2001 Harper-Collins Publishers. Fortunately for everybody, modern medicine is beginning to catch up with the healing wisdom of the Maya and other ancient cultures.

Numerous studies have underlined the link between high blood pressure, arthritis, heart disease, asthma, bronchitis and even cancer with unresolved emotional stress and distress.

At the same time an array of studies in neuroscience also explain how brain chemistry affects our mental and emotional states. That's because the mind and the body are directly connected.

Suddenly, as if it's something new psychotherapists and medical doctors are once again being taught to consider the importance of the mind and body connection in disease treatment.

Near Vera Cruz Mexico, Olmec civilization emerged around 1200-900 B.C. The Olmec are considered the mother of Meso American civilizations. Maya villages are thought to have begun forming around 1000 B.C.

The population grew, eventually spreading into what is now Belize, Guatemala, western parts of Honduras and El Salvador and the Yucatan, Tabasco and Chiapas in Mexico.

The Maya began to build cities and to distinguish themselves in writing, art, astronomy, engineering and architecture. Maya architectural, astronomical, mathematical and engineering feats have fascinated us for generations.

But very few people are aware of their sophisticated and effective medical system. Anthropologists consider Mayan medicine a medical religious system. In essence the Mayans have a two pronged approach to healing.

They have remedies for a wide range of plaguing physical ailments that any individual or health practitioner would be pleased to add to a health repertoire.

As part of the visible world, physical ailments like stomach aches, heart issues or infected wounds are handled with natural empirical or naturalistic knowledge.

The Mayans have equally effective remedies, however for the ailments of the spirit that the human eye cannot see, such as sadness, grief, fright and envy. They are part of the magical mystical world and have traditionally been the responsibility of the h'men.

The heh man is another word for healer, doctor, priest or shaman. Mayan healers believe that these ailments involving the soul and spirits are supernatural in origin and these supernatural forces can both sicken and heal.

The natural and supernatural bodies of knowledge are intertwined. For example, Mayan plant lore does not exist in a state of separation from the human soul. This concept is sometimes difficult for the modern mind trained in separatist ideology to grasp.

The union of these two worlds allows Mayan medicine to go beyond modern medicine. Over the years I have begun to discover the magical side of Mayan medicine extremely useful for both my patients and myself.

The Mayan paradigm has opened doors that I never knew existed. Their ideas about spiritual illness have helped me understand why some people get well and some people do not, even when their illnesses are the same.

Traditional healing is a tapestry that has been woven by humans throughout history. The patterns reverberate from culture to culture and the themes are universal.

Mayan healers can use plants, stones, animals, water and especially prayers to heal.

At the very heart of Mayan medicine is the concept that medicine is all around us. We pass it daily right on our very doorstep. We also find it at roadsides and in trees, plants, stones, animals, dreams and prayers. The earth mother is the source of medicinal power.

Basic Tools Of Mayan Healing

The Mayan view of the human condition is extremely broad. A Mayan healer would never expect someone to recover simply by talking out a problem, changing his or her behavior or environment or through simply taking an oral medication.

Although they do use these tools, their medicine chest has more to offer. Prayer first and foremost, the sastun which is a stone or crystal used by the h'men to communicate with:

-The Mayan spirits

-Medicinal plants

-Herbal baths

-Incense

-Holy water

-Dream visions

-Rituals and ceremony

-Amulets

Prayer

Whenever I ask a Mayan healer of any age "What is your most important healing tool?" they always answer with a single word "Prayer." Prayer is at the heart of the Mayan medical religious system and is used by all traditional healers, whether snake doctor or midwife.

It is the prayer that carries the ch'ulel which is a vibrant energy force that the Mayans believe emanates from a divine spiritual source between the physical and spiritual worlds.

One of the main goals of Mayan healing is to balance the flow of ch'ulel that flows in and out of the body. Prayers are intrinsically powerful verbal sounds that embody the power of God. To recite that power is to know it.

A power residing in each individual, prayer is tapped through meditation and rituals. Prayer unites the individual with the universal, the physical with the divine and allows us to both give and receive love.

Mayan prayers are very similar to the medicine songs of North American indigenous people. They are chants repeated nine times in a soft whisper. The prayers are always repeated nine times.

Three prayers are said while holding the patients right radial pulse at the wrist, then three at the left radial pulse and finally three more while placing both hands over the top of the skull and forehead, which the Mayans believe to be the fountain of the spirit.

Prayers must be said with faith. Faith is the foundation on which all else is built in Mayan medicine. This shouldn't be big news. Study after study has shown that there is a relationship between faith and the immune system.

Medicinal Plants

The Mayan word for medicinal plant is xiv (sheev). Xiv is either primary medicine in the form of vines, roots or barks or secondary medicine from leaves and flowers.

Thousands of medicinal plants are available to the Mayan healer, but each healer settles on two dozen that he or she uses daily. Healers may use others as the need arises.

The choice of plants depends upon the kinds of ailments being treated. Plants are collected with respect, reverence and prayer. Like all of the earth's resources, plants are imbued with ch'ulel, which must be engaged so that the plant acts with full potency.

When you say the prayer of thanksgiving and faith to the plant, the plant spirit follows you home to help with the healing. Without a prayer, the spiritual essence of the plant returns to the earth and the healing is at its best, random chance.

It is also important to have faith in the plants healing propensities. When you go out to gather medicinal plants don't say "I hope this will work out" or "Maybe this will work." Clearly state your faith that it will work.

Medicinal plants can be prepared as teas, made into tinctures in alcohol, steeped in oil to produce a healing salve for the skin, dried and powdered for wounds, boiled with sugar to make syrups, mashed with salt to make poultices and administered as herbal baths.

Medicinal plants can also be dried, powdered and rolled into cornhusks and smoked. But you must remember that when smoking anything, there are side effects that come from inhaling any smoke.

Pulses

Every Mayan healer starts by checking the patients pulse. The conduit of the body's ch'ulel, the pulsing blood provides information about the physical and spiritual condition of the patient. The Maya go far beyond the modern medical system's use of the pulse.

Medical doctors count the number of pulse beats per minute, but Mayan healers recognize eighteen different kinds of pulses. They listen for strength, depth, rapidity, rhythm, location and bounce.

Herbal Baths

If the lost art of therapeutic herbal bathing were to be rediscovered, a very useful tool would be restored to healers and physicians. Hydrotherapy and sea water therapy have been part of the fabric of medicine since the earliest of times.

The Mayans consider water ch'ulel. It is an elixir that refreshes and purifies the body. Herbal baths combine the power of water with that of plants. Together they absorb our pain, fear and anxiety and leave us cleansed and renewed at a deep energetic level.

When plants are collected and prepared with prayer and loving intent, an additional energy charge is transmitted to the patient.

Massage

Nearly all Mayan healers incorporate therapeutic touch and massage into their treatment of both spiritual and physical ailments.

Counseling

Who can live without someone to talk to in times of need? The healers become intuitive experts at compassionate listening and giving good common sense advice.

An encouraging word, a sympathetic ear, a shared story and a pat on the back can mean so much. A loving word is to the afflicted what sun and rain are to the earth.

Humor

Many healers use humor. Humor is the best tool a healer can have in his or her bag. Most people think too much, but get them to laugh and half of their trouble and sickness will go away.

Ritual And Ceremony

A good healing ritual can make people feel better. The Mayans include ritual in almost every aspect of their healing system. When a healer doesn't know what else to do, a simple ritual of prayer, bathing and incense can seem close to miraculous.

Incense

Incense is the essence of life, the scent of the spirit. Certain resins and dried parts of sacred plants release ch'ulel when burned. The resin of the copal tree is collected with ritual and ceremony on full moon nights.

Bits of copal are dropped onto a bed of coals. Copal is burned for the treatment of all spiritual diseases, improves mood and is also considered helpful for many physical ailments.

The belief is that the copal incense can rid a person of a harmful or improper thought process, cleanse a home of fear and envy and act as an offering to the Gods and Goddesses.

In addition to copal, the Maya also burn dried rosemary leaves and powdered balsam bark. Whatever remedies you try, be sure to use common sense at all times. Watch for side effects, and be alert for allergic reactions.

Be aware ahead of time of possible interactions between herbs and drugs and always remain in touch with your physician. Mayan medical wisdom is an additional perspective, not a replacement for visiting your health care provider.

THE SCALPEL AND THE SILVER BEAR

Let us continue on our journey of examining aspects of healing from different cultures. The more people I meet and talk with, the more I learn. Another learning adventure has been with assistance from my friend Wilma Lawrence.

Wilma grew up on the "Rez" at Red Lake. We met at the United Theological Seminary and as we got to know each other we began to discuss our journeys and discoveries on the path of spirituality and healing.

Wilma shared with me "The Scalpel and the Silver Bear" by Lori Arviso Alvord M.D. and Elizabeth Cohen Van Pelt from Bantam Books. Lori's father was Navajo and her mother Anglo. She grew up in Crown Point, New Mexico with two cultures.

She attended Dartmouth and received her medical training at Stanford University Medical School. The book describes her struggles to bring modern medicine to the

Navajo reservation in Gallup and to bring the values of her people to a medical care system.

Navajo people have a concept called Walking in Beauty, but it isn't the beauty that most people think of. Beauty to Navajos means living in balance and harmony with yourself and the world.

It means caring for yourself, mind, body and spirit and having the right relationships with your family, community, the animal world, the environment, earth, air, water, our planet and our universe.

If a person respects and honors all these relationships then they will be walking in beauty. For Navajos, healers and holy men were merged and doctors and priests were one in the same, they did not isolate a part from the whole.

Their medicine was for the whole human creature, body, mind and spirit, their community and even the larger world. The world heal comes from the same root as whole and holiness. For Navajos, wholeness and holiness is the same thing.

The system of life is one interconnected whole. Everything is related. The causes and cures for illness are woven into everything else. A Navajo healer will look at the person's whole life and the lives around the person.

A person might be sick because he treats his wife, children or elders unkindly or has a bad attitude towards his neighbors or has neglected his body and become lazy and fat.

He may be too absorbed in acquiring wealth or other personal gains and has neglected those around him. A Navajo healer will look for the imbalance. The stress from disharmony can cause physical sickness, depression, even violence and death.

If the concept of balance is extended to the community level, then communities out of balance will have problems such as gang violence, elder neglect, child abuse and drug use.

As Western society moves to a focus on the individual rather than the community, the support of the community has faded away. Apply this same concept to the national level and it is clear that if nations do not live in harmony together, then wars are a natural result.

Now in the nuclear age, the health of all humanity weighs in the balance. An imbalance of humans with the natural world also leads to illness. While it may seem obvious, an imbalance in the natural world can have disastrous consequences.

Native people have always been careful to respect the animal world. Many tribes feel that humans are not superior to animals and that animals have spirits as well.

Living in balance with the rest of the animal world has protected species for millennia, but western society doesn't share the view that this is essential. Now many species are being exterminated by humans, either deliberately or as a result of carelessness.

It is hard for native people to believe that humans can be so uncaring as to wipe another species off the face of the earth, but it is happening all around us now.

And it is not only the animal world that is under attack, but the environment as well. In time, since we live in a closely interrelated ecosystem, one of these careless acts could backfire and put the human species itself at risk for extinction.

Human health is dependent upon planetary health. All must exist in a delicate web of balanced relationships. Little has been written or can be shared by Native American healers.

The medicine is passed on by living and doing. The translation of the language and culture to western ways and English is sadly lacking and there is no word for that in English.

Healing is sacred and not to be misused. It is holy and not to be taken at all in a frivolous way. And it must come from a deep understanding and acceptance of self and environment.

"Honoring the Medicine" by Kenneth Cohen is A One World Book Published by The Random House Ballantine Publishing Company, is a collection of information about Native American medicine and a healing philosophy that connects each of us with the whole web of life.

An excerpt from Honoring the Medicine states that Native American healing is America's original holistic medicine. Native American healing emphasizes harmony with the earth as an essential ingredient in personal health.

But how can we find harmony with the earth if we continue to cut her hair (the forests), steal her bones (minerals) and dump poisons into her blood stream (rivers and oceans)?

We cannot preserve the original healing traditions without recognizing the rights of the people of North America, into autonomy and control over their own lives and lands.

The elders say that plants, swimmers, crawlers, four legged, and those who fly are also people with God given rights to the food, shelter and happiness that nature provides.

The objectivity of science is a euphemism that often masks unconscious, culture bound preconceptions about the criteria that determine truth. Native American healing goes far beyond the boundaries or capabilities of science.

To accurately measure the effectiveness of Native American healing, a researcher would have to measure not only physiological or biochemical improvements but also changes in the patient's happiness and the well being of his or her family and community.

Learning to become a traditional healer is hard work. It requires years of rigorous training and testing and consistent demonstration of endurance, courage, patience, generosity and in general character.

Humor is also an essential ingredient. Elders will not teach people who take themselves too seriously or who become disheartened in the face of suffering. Nor will they train a lazy person.

Native American healers are unified in their belief that the Great Spirit is the source of healing and life. The terms Great Spirit, Great Mystery, Creator and God are interchangeable.

Many consider the Great Spirit beyond or inclusive of all genders and may thus use masculine and or feminine forms of address. The Great Spirit is the creator of all life.

Because the Great Spirit formed all life out of the same elements, human beings are interconnected and related to nature. A harmonious relationship with nature promotes health, while living out of balance with the web of life promotes illness.

Prayer is communication with the Great Spirit and/ or the wise beings or powers that the Great Spirit created and it includes both listening and speaking. To pray to the Great Spirit is to seek unity with the Great Spirit. It is good to begin and end each day with prayer.

Pray before eating and before all important activities. A spiritual person embodies spiritual values such as honesty, honor, respect, humility, courage, patience, generosity and humor. A spiritual person inspires and teaches these values by example.

He or she has what Native Americans call a "Good Mind." Native Americans understand that both humor and mystical insight arise from a flexible consciousness and the ability to perceive in a new way or from multiple perspectives.

Flexibility is also the essence of harmonious relationships and conflict resolution. When people ask me "What is Native American spirituality ?" I usually discuss the Cycles of Truth.

The Cycles Of Truth is a twelve pointed medicine wheel like the face of a clock that represents fundamental Native American values. These values are the foundation of integrity or wholeness, balance and happiness.

The Cycles of Truth clearly show that Native American spirituality is not a matter of doing this or that ceremony or wearing buckskin and beating a drum, but is rather a state of mind and heart. It is very simply being a good person and living in harmony with nature.

The values represented on the Cycles of Truth are generally called "gifts." In contrast to the Christian assumption of original sin, Native Americans believe that all people are born with spiritual values that are gifts from the creator.

To Native Americans people are not born with original sin, but with original sanctity. Native American spirituality models virtuous behavior rather than restricting bad behavior. There is no Native American equivalent to the Ten Commandments.

Instead of saying "Thou shall not covet," Native elders say "An honorable person is generous." Native Americans focus upon prescribing states of mind, the states of mind to be attained in a progression toward an ultimate self realization.

The elders' teachings are meant to awaken our innate goodness which means that a person who attains higher spiritual state will naturally behave in a morally positive direction.

Implicit in this philosophy is the notion that Native American values are not rules that must be obeyed but rather good words that are meant to inspire, guide and instruct. Elders who teach values by modeling them "walk the walk."

The 12 Cycles Of Truth

<u>LEARNING</u>. Learning requires balance and open mindedness, silence and awareness. Elders stress the importance of observation, listening and patience rather than the questioning and analysis that are the hallmarks of Western education.

Questioning for the sake of clarification or to clear up a misunderstanding is good, but we must be careful not to stunt our own problem solving ability or survival by asking questions too soon. In Native American culture, learning is cooperative and interactive.

<u>HONORING</u>. Honor is the respect for the creator, creation, yourself and others. It means both self esteem and esteeming others because we are the children of the Great Spirit.

With honor we respect our differences including religious and spiritual ones. Elders across Indian

America agree that respect is the foundation of a happy and satisfying life.

<u>ACCEPTANCE</u>. The gift of acceptance means seeing and acknowledging the spiritual beauty in all beings and appreciating them for what they are rather than trying to manipulate or mold them into what one would like them to be.

Acceptance also means not being a perfectionist and forgiving the faults we see in ourselves and others. It is important that we accept our weaknesses even as we know our strengths.

Without doing so we are likely to ignore our problems or to blame others, making it more difficult to change or improve. Acceptance is not blind or passive. It has limits. We should seek to change any situation that is harmful or unjust.

The gift of acceptance is thus balanced by "responsibility" and the ability to respond appropriately with fortitude, courage, wisdom and compassion.

<u>SEEING</u>. The gift of seeing is spiritual insight which is defined as:

The ability to perceive subtle or hidden truths with the eye of the spirit. This gives you the ability to view life from a higher and wider perspective. And helps one to realize that all events in our lives are connected in mysterious and meaningful ways.

<u>HEARING</u>. The gift of hearing means sensitivity to the vibrations or energy of life, with a clear minded receptivity. The gift of hearing means sensitivity to the vibrations of all kinds of sound frequencies. Like words, music and other forms of sound.

<u>SPEAKING</u>. The gift of speaking is connected to the gift of hearing. It is important to speak from our listening

and to speak with a quiet, humble and open mind whether we are communicating with people or nature.

A basic rule of traditional Indian oratory is never to try to coerce or persuade other people into believing your own truth. Speak with strength but without arrogance and If your words are true listeners will accept them.

If you try to compel belief, listeners will mistrust your message. Speaking is communicating with the Great Spirit in prayer and with the spirits of stones, plants and animals. Many Native American traditions say sound is a creative force.

When something is named, its being is evoked. To say wind is to call on the power of the wind. This is especially true of indigenous languages because they are direct expressions of the land from which they arose.

Words are carried by sacred breath. They have power and always must be spoken with care. Hurtful thoughts and words may have harmful consequences and loving words can heal.

<u>LOVING</u>. Loving is love of the Great Spirit and love of the earth and all who dwell upon her. Its symbol is the sun. The sun shines on all unconditionally and it is always present even when we can't see it.

Love gives meaning to life yet we cannot create or attract it intentionally. Love is not a matter of effort, it comes as a grace when we prepare ourselves day by day by living in a good way. The human mind divides subject from object and thus exiles us from nature.

Love reminds us that happiness is found when we surrender to forces that are unknown and unknowable. Native healers use the power of love in their work.

We were instructed to carry a love for one another and to show great respect for all the beings of this earth. In other words, love and respect are the essence of the creators original instructions.

<u>SERVICE</u>. The elders teach us to serve community and to do what is necessary to preserve the mental, physical, spiritual and environmental health of family and neighbors.

Service also means generosity which is one of the cardinal virtues in Indian Country. There are two kinds of wealth. First wealth is having a big family and many relations.

The second kind of wealth might sound paradoxical from a non Native perspective. A wealthy person may have few possessions and little money because true wealth is not measured by how much you accumulate but by how much and how often you give.

A person who shares resources and helps those in need is a rich and honorable person. Generosity may be a necessity for profound healing and is necessary for a person to feel connected to the universe and God.

<u>LIVING</u>. It is not enough to know and speak the truth, we must live it put it into action. Living the truth implies deliberate, focused action and balanced use of the minds power to focus. Set noble goals in your life and then do your best to accomplish them.

The earth supports and nurtures all forms and stages of life and teaches observant people to do the same. The mother earth is a role model of unconditional caring and living in balance.

<u>WORKING</u>. Work means far more than earning money or "making a living." It involves the hands, the mind, the heart and the cooperation of others. In the Wolf Clan Teaching Lodge work is symbolized by the turtle.

The turtle does everything slowly and carefully. His pace is dictated by the rhythms of nature. He is on "Indian time". Things get done when they need to get done. No schedules or clocks.

<u>WALKING</u>. "Walking the truth" means walking in a spiritual path through life and remaining in motion which means realizing that spirituality is dynamic rather than passive. To Native Americans, walking was more than recreation or exercise, it's a matter of survival.

To walk is to appreciate and learn from the landscape and to discover the location of building and craft materials and edible plants and animals. To walk a spiritual trial is to walk with courage and commitment. Walk your vision and walk your goals.

<u>GRATITUDE</u>. The simplest and profoundest Native American prayer is to say "Thank you" four or seven times. When Native people pray they do not say "I want, give me" but "I offer" and "I am grateful."

Gratefulness is a free expression of the heart. We need to develop our twelve gifts in order to have a prosperous, happy, purposeful, beautiful and to live a meaningful and joyous life.

THE HEALING WISDOM
OF AFRICA

Let us continue our journey of exploring other perspectives of healing and spirituality. In the book Healing Wisdom of Africa: Finding Life Purpose Through Nature, Ritual and Community (©1998 Jeremy P. Tarcher/Putnam) Malidoma.

Patrice comes from a little village in West Africa named Dano, located in Burkina Faso (formerly Upper Volta). He is a gifted initiated diviner and medicine man of the Dagara tribe.

He holds three masters degree's and two doctorates from the Sorbonne and Brandeis.The Dagara people are well known throughout West Africa for beliefs and practices that outsiders find both fascinating and frightening.

The Dagara connection with beings from the spirit world has resulted in the accumulation of first hand knowledge of subjects regarded in the west as paranormal, magical or spiritual.

Dagara "science" in this sense is the investigation of the spirit world. What in the west might be regarded as fiction, among the Dagara is believed as fact for we have seen it with our eyes, heard it with our ears or felt it with our own hands.

The stories I tell often sounds to western ears as unbelievable. It's because they lack the advantage of the comprehensive investigations into the interplay of spirit and matter that characterize the Dagara and many other African peoples.

At the colonial school I have been told that the rituals my people performed to heal were devilish or satanic. At school we had been also told that tribal people had no knowledge of magic but instead were very superstitious.

When I witnessed Dagara people make things appear and disappear into thin air and when I witnessed beings from the Other World show up in flesh and bones allowing me to touch them, I wondered how superstitious all this was.

And then there was my introduction to the Kontombli who are the spirits in the wild who worked as the comforter of every person in need. All of these experiences contradicted the theories disseminated in the schools.

At the same time it was interesting to see the reactions of villagers who observed what literacy had done to me. I discovered that from their perspective what I learned from my white teachers was considered poison and even dangerous to myself and others.

It was as if literacy destroyed the ability to learn the indigenous knowledge that I was trying to reclaim. With literacy had come a logic that was incompatible with the logic innate to the Dagara and other native peoples.

It made me prone to doubt, incapable of trust and subject to dangerous emotions such as anger and impatience. Worst of all, my western perceptions of time were continually disturbing me in a culture in which timelessness prevailed.

For an African to come to the west while maintaining a devotion to ancestral wisdom is to invoke a program of challenges and adversity. Here in the West, Africa has been much written about.

But in areas such as religion and spirituality where Africa has quite a profound wisdom to contribute, it has been for the most part written off. Many Westerners have written about African spirituality, but they pay no attention to the practices that might benefit Westerners.

Most references instead discuss rather disturbing magical practices such as blood sacrifices, voodoo and witch doctors involved in evil rituals. And in fact, scores of educated Africans in positions of influence have publicly rejected the spiritual practices of their kinfolk.

They consider their practices as primitive and barbaric. I found here in the west people who were so submerged in the massive trance of modern culture that they appeared virtually unreachable.

It became clear that certain topics of discussion, such as spirituality and rituals were not permitted in intellectual and professional circles. They are often rejected because of their comfort with their new ways of thinking.

I noticed some people, particularly those who were the most enthralled by the game of consumerism, found mentions of indigenous wisdom especially irritating and would sometimes lash out at me.

I am still recovering from the anger, irritation and inflamed words of the people who retaliated at me, just for referring to the indigenous people as having a great power.

I have gradually come to understand that one thing Western and indigenous people share is the fact that both have elected to live here on earth and are thus subject to the spirit of earth.

By this I simply mean that indigenous and western people are actually children of the same spirit, living in the same house they call earth. No matter what they do to torture each other, the dysfunctional relationship of modern and indigenous people is symptomatic.

Symptomatic of a craving to share love for each other that is deeply buried in our psyche, a craving so alive that it is compelled to struggle through the rubble of division, power conflicts and fear to express itself.

What the indigenous world offers to the modern world centers around the understanding of the concepts of healing, ritual and community. Indigenous communities have since time immemorial focused their lives and their existence on these issues.

Healing is central because it was learned very early that human beings are vulnerable to psychological and biological breakdown and that this general instability touches all aspects of their existence.

They have also learned that the natural environment in which they live is made up of subtle invisible things that if manipulated in certain ways can affect the conditions that they intended to heal. Ritual is the technology that allows the manipulation of these subtle energies.

Community is important because there is an understanding that human beings are collectively oriented. The general health and well being of an individual are connected to a community and are not something that can be maintained alone or in a vacuum.

Healing, ritual and community, these three elements are virtually linked. Indigenous people see the physical world as a reflection of a more complex, subtler and more lasting yet invisible entity called energy.

It is as if we are the shadows of a vibrant and endlessly resourceful intelligence dynamically involved in a process of continuous self creation. Nothing happens here that did not begin in that unseen world.

If something in the physical world is experiencing instability, it is because of its energetic correspondent has been experiencing instability. They are both correlated to each other.

The indigenous understanding is that the material and physical problems that a person encounters are important only because they are an energetic message sent to this visible world.

Therefore people go to that unseen energetic place to try to repair any damage or disturbances that are being done there, knowing that if things are healed there, things will be healed there.

Ritual is the principle tool used to approach that unseen world in a way that will rearrange the structure of the physical world and bring about material transformation. Connecting with the unseen realities made visible in our symbols is crucial to the well being of our psyches.

 A person who walks through a ritual and ends up feeling charged and invigorated is a blessed recipient of healing waves of energy that no one can see but everyone can benefit from.

The full heart of a person blessed in this manner overflows into the needy souls of others, igniting the healing fire most wanted for self replenishment. Ritual is essential to village life.

Because rituals provide the focus and the energy that holds the community together. And they also provide the kind of healing that the community needs the most to survive.

Because healing in the indigenous world includes the dimensions of the spirit, definitions of illness extend also to the unseen worlds of mind and spirit. The inability to perceive and the inability to understand to indigenous people are symptomatic of an illness.

If your psyche is disordered, deficient or over charged, there are blocks that are created in you that prevent comprehension and remembering. To open up the channels in you so that whatever energy you need can flow freely is not the task of the teacher, it is the task of the shaman.

Another form of this illness is the inability to accept or even tolerate those who are different from us. Worse, this inability encourages suspicion, fear and resentment.

Thus, it is an illness of the collective psyche when different cultures don't understand one another.

The history of humankind is plagued by this disease that has caused much pain and disappointment in the world. Methods of healing must take into account the energetic or spiritual condition that is in turmoil, thereby affecting the physical condition.

If you focus only on the physical translation of the underlying energetic disorder, then you are ignoring the true source of the physical illness. You are ignoring the cause of the problem.

If you address only the physical problem, then you may end up with a cure that fixes the physical condition, providing only a momentary sense of victory over debilitation.

But this act denies the needs of the energy, the adjustment of the spirit needed to make the cure last.

Sooner or later this disordered energy will figure out a new way to affect the physical body often in a new and more virulent manner than it did originally.

If you instead address the energy of the mind and Spirit whose status is affecting the physical body, then you are likely to truly heal. Hence, in the wisdom of indigenous concepts of healing, all healing must begin by first addressing the energetic problems.

Once a person addresses the energetic problem, then rituals are used. Because rituals involved in removing the energetic problem is where the transformation and healing occurs.

If something comes into our lives and we deny it by labeling it impossible, an indigenous elder would interpret this way of thinking as a manifestation of our own rigidity in the face of new possibilities.

In the mind of a villager, the unreal is just a new and yet unconfirmed reality in the vocabulary of consciousness. It is brought to us by the ancestors. A little hospitality towards it will suffice, to make it part of us.

In short, the indigenous mind does not admit impossibility. It defines itself by not rejecting the unfamiliar and it therefore thrives on mysteries and magic.

Such a mind gives ample space to the invisible because the invisible holds the key to the wisdom of the universe. A physical body alone cannot have any sort of direction in this life.

So it is important to recognize that the body is an extension of the spirit and the spirit is an extension of the body. The two are inseparable. This is nothing supernatural, it is just what is.

The Cosmos As A Wheel

In Dagara cosmology the image and structure of the circle or wheel organizes perceptions of the world. The wheel not only refers to the cyclic nature of life, but it is also a microcosm of the circular nature of the planet where we live.

The indigenous tendency is to perceive all of life within the context of this circular cycle or cosmology. When something of cosmic proportion occurs, such as an earthquake, plague or drought, seeing it as a part of a wheel determines the approach and attitude towards it.

In the West by contrast, where progress is seen as a linear journey into the future, a natural catastrophe is approached as an unfortunate obstacle. The reaction is to fix the problem by removing the obstacle and then move on.

The results are regarded as damage or cost and are measured in terms of dollars and cents. The event is seen as an attack or an insurgency that must be quickly countered, stepped over and relegated to the past of a linear history.

For example, an earthquake in Los Angeles that downs bridges and homes is quickly answered by an almost instant rebuilding. It is as if people cannot tolerate the directness of Mother Earth's message to us.

It must be erased quickly as possible, because it comes as interference to the forward motion of civilization. This is a logical reaction to a linear view of life. An indigenous African interpretation would be that the shaking of the earth is a message to us.

We may not understand it at first, but we must come down to our knees with prayers of consternation and mourning while expressing the willingness to understand that this event in the natural world and our lives are connected.

Meanwhile village life is suspended until all prescribed rituals are done. Then reconstruction, if appropriate can begin in peace. This approach is based on an understanding of the cyclical nature of life.

In this cyclical nature of life, everything that exists in time and space, the earth, moon and other planets is part of a continuous wheel and is connected to everything that happens.

An event that is not addressed properly, that is cosmologically bound to happen in a more forceful tone because it needs to be understood and adequately replied to and not silenced or ignored.

This is why cosmology is the key to indigenous life and spirituality. I have been using names such as water people, fire people, earth people, mineral people and nature people. Indeed these five elements are also definable by clan.

People are born into one or another of the clans, much like being born under a certain astrological sign. It is the time of your birth that stamps the element it carries on you.

The decision of when to be born and which element to embody is considered by indigenous people to be prenatal and is sealed by the individual. The five elements which make up five clans allow the entire village to form a cosmological wheel.

The village can then balance itself by keeping the various elements in balance. For the wheel to be balanced there must be an overwhelming representation of water.

Just as the earth is essentially water and just as the human body is essentially water, a community needs a large number of water people to maintain its balance. There must be at least three times more people of water in the village than people of fire.

When there are not, symbolic heat creeps in and rises, resulting in crisis. The difficulty of forming community in the modern world seems to arise from this, for when the people coming together are predominantly of fire friction is produced more often than balance.

This is why there are healing rituals aimed at coping with problems of energetic imbalance. Water rituals can help calm the fire and produce reconciliation with nature.

Indeed, when the proportion of water is more than three times that of fire, the earth becomes moist enough for nature to flourish. Water feeds nature, so the presence of water results in vitality, growing plant and animal life.

A healthy relationship of water, earth and nature will result in clean air to breathe. When these three elements are not in balance, the air we breathe is poor in quality. To upset the balance of elements is to throw the community into danger.

The principal task of a community is to maintain balance. A state in which all five elements are functioning smoothly, echoing one another. To achieve this requires great diligence on the part of a community.

This effort need not be undertaken through the application of sophisticated theories of economic or social welfare. It is first necessary to determine which elements are troubling the community.

The elemental wheel exists in each person just as it is present in each clan and in every community. This means that each person on a smaller scale must maintain a state of balance at all cost.

Each person needs to keep the waters of reconciliation flowing within the self in order to calm the inner fires and live in harmony with others. Each person needs to nourish the ancestral fire within, so that one stays in touch with ones dreams and visions.

Each person needs to be grounded in the earth, to be able to become a source of nourishment to the community. Each person needs to remember the knowledge stored in one's bones, and to live out one's own unique genius.

And each person needs to be real, as nature is real, that is without pretense, keeping in touch with a sense of mystery and wonder and helping to preserve the integrity of the natural world.

To be out of balance in any of these areas is to invite sickness to come dwell within. A person who is out of balance threatens to throw the entire community out of balance.

In the village, the illness of any one person calls forth the energy of the entire community. If any individual is sick, then the village is sick. A community is healthy when everybody in it is healthy.

The fire of a person who is in an emotional crisis can easily expand out to other people and before the problem is identified, the entire community could be ablaze. In the modern world ideological or dogmatic thought can be quite dangerous in a similar way.

Ideology and dogma contain an elemental fiery energy of a distinct signature that can surge. Without protective efforts, the surging energy can spread to other circuits and enflame a whole system, a whole culture.

Individual healing can be seen as a protection of life's energetic wheel, for only when all of the individuals in a community are healthy can there be health in the community itself.

THANK YOU FOR READING

If You Received Useful Tools In This Information, Please Give Me A 4-5 Star Rating!

This serves as a reward for an author. It takes hours and months, sometimes years of no pay to put together books for the purpose of sharing information you see as important to the world.

Please just take out a minute of your time and please leave a quick positive review. Thank you tremendously for taking out the time to read this information and knowledge.

If you really took this information seriously and you applied the key principles into your daily life, I KNOW you are seeing results.

So again, I thank you for your interest in learning and any investment in applied knowledge will always be a winning investment.

For More Books By

Rev. Dr. Geraldine L. Johnson-Carter Visit:

amazon.com/author/geraldinejohnsoncarter